Detoxification: A guide for medically assisted withdrawal from chemical addiction in the residential setting

CW01046416

Detoxification: A guide for medically assisted withdrawal from chemical addiction in the residential setting

by

Dr Gordon R Morse

Quay
Books

Quay Books Division, Mark Allen Publishing Group, Jesses Farm, Snow Hill, Dinton, Salisbury, Wiltshire SP3 5HN

British Library Cataloguing-in-Publication Data
A catalogue record is available for this book

© Dr Gordon R Morse 1999
ISBN 1 85642 177 5

Printed in the UK by Antony Rowe Ltd, Chippenham

Contents

Acknowledgements

This book is pooled from the knowledge, experience and wisdom of everyone whom I count myself lucky to have worked with at Clouds. From my predecessor Dr Erica Douglas, from David Marteau and our team of nurses, from Paul Sunderland, and from Chris Peberdy and his team of counsellors. Every one of these remarkable and caring people has a breadth and depth of knowledge in this highly specialised field which I have drawn upon from time to time.

Finally, having overseen more than a thousand treatments, I must thank the patients themselves. The survivors who I see at reunions and those that I do not.

These are all extraordinary people, there isn't one who hasn't moved me in some way and taught me in another. The learning process continues for me on a daily basis, and I am very grateful to all of them for making this book possible, and my life a fuller one.

Gordon R Morse
March, 1999

Foreword

Chemical abuse varies widely in severity, from the social drinker whose intake sometimes exceeds acceptable safe limits to the heroin addict with a daily intravenous habit of a couple of grammes as well as frequent pipes of crack cocaine, washed down with several cans of high-octane lager. For the former, some health education may suffice; for the latter, a completely different approach may be called for: in-patient 'primary' treatment with a view to sustained abstinence.

Such a radical change of lifestyle may be unnecessary for many people who have experienced substance difficulties, yet for others it would appear to be the only realistic way to avoid certain self-destruction. For these unlucky few alcohol and other drugs have a near paralysing effect on the will so that control is never regained.

The abstinence treatment approach has grown from the disease model of addiction — the notion that sufferers are in some way 'allergic' to mind affecting chemicals, and the compulsion to consume them follows a chronic and ultimately disastrous trend. This paradigm is not without its critics. Barber for instance, pointed out an inherent contradiction in the argument: that the answer to an illness symptomised by an inability to control substance use, is the control of substance use. Viewed this way, the abstinence movement appears to be based on philosophical sleight of hand, yet I have known many people who are convinced that it has saved their lives.

Perhaps in response to this criticism, Alcoholics Anonymous use the aphorism:

'I alone can do it, but I can't do it alone.'

Paradox is a common component of addiction. It is baffling for instance, that the condition afflicts many people of above average intelligence who seem unable to make the simple calculation, 'This is plainly dangerous, I will stop'.

Others have argued that since a problem of dependence generally centres on a single drug, avoidance of just that drug of choice is a viable solution. Total abstinence appears abhorrent, even puritanical to some critics. This issue is frequently debated at Clouds. Recently, in response to the question from a heroin addict 'Why am I not allowed to still have an (alcoholic) drink now and again?' A fellow patient in the group answered, 'I am an alcoholic. Do you think it would be OK for me to use heroin now and again?' As Dr John Marks has pointed out, the legality of a substance is no indicator of its safety.

Another common theme in our work with dependency is the historic belief that alcoholics and drug addicts are liars. They are not. However, faced with a potentially difficult situation, someone in the grip of an addiction will tend to avoid the risk of pain or punishment: 'I only had one','No, I haven't seen your purse', 'I dropped the bottle and it broke'.

Thomas Szasz was probably right when he said that any person is only as honest as he or she can afford to be. To be honest about one's addiction is to accept its presence and power, and in so doing, to countenance separation from a loyal (albeit dangerous) chemical companion.

In part, and only in part, chemical dependency may represent the translation of emotional and psychological need, into desire. In detoxification, unsatisfied need may exacerbate physical discomfort. Revising a contracted detoxification regime can be detrimental to a patient's best interests, should a doctor endeavour to extinguish each somatised symptom.

I have never known Gordon Morse yield to this temptation and I am delighted to say that he probably never will. To defeat addiction, courage is required on the part of the physician as well as the patient. Often the most considerate response is 'No', and Gordon Morse has become referred to by his patients with some respect and (interestingly) some affection, as 'Dr No'.

David Marteau
Co-ordinator of the treatment team
Clouds House
March 1998

References

Barber JG (1995) *Social Work with Addicts*, Macmillan, Basingstoke

Marks J (1997) from a speech given in Paris, *The Economic and Social Costs of Public Drug Dependency Policies*

Szasz T (1961) *The Myth of Mental Illness*. Harper and Row, London

Preface

The morning after the first night that I arrived in Dundee to start my medical education in October 1971, I awoke to the news that someone had been stabbed on my Hall doorstep in what was described later in the press as a 'drug-related' incident. My five years at that excellent Scottish teaching hospital was spent treating enormous numbers of patients whose medical condition was complicated by, or often solely caused by, alcohol abuse. Indeed, it was the policy of some Consultants to commence every patient admitted on high dose vitamin B supplements, on the assumption that every citizen of Dundee was an alcoholic until proven otherwise. Yet I do not recall a single lecture on the subject of chemical abuse in the whole time I was studying to become a doctor.

But it would be quite wrong to single out my medical school in this way, for asking around my colleagues in the years since, it seems that this continues to be a widespread omission from the education of healthworkers, doctors and nurses alike. And omission it is, a massive one. Alcohol and drug abuse (I shall simplify the nomenclature to 'chemical abuse') impacts on the lives of enormous numbers of people around the world. The UK is as typical as most countries with 2.5% of the entire population drinking regularly above the WHO guidelines, at least 300,000 dependent on opiates, and an estimated 400,000 doses of Ecstasy taken every single week. Quite apart from the causation of disease or even death to the individual, chemical abuse damages our society: it leads directly to prostitution, unemployment, burglary, assaults, a burgeoning prison population, divorce, child abuse, and funds organised crime. In so doing, it creates misery and from misery springs the drive to palliate the misery. Abuse breeds abuse, and chemical abuse breeds chemical abuse, a cycle of social, physical and emotional disease.

Much has been written about chemical abuse, most of it excellent work that will aid understanding and empower health workers to make a real contribution to the lives of those who have been affected. Most of this work centres on understanding the patient's psychodynamics; how corruption of emotional development creates a 'valency' for chemical abuse, and how helping the patient to identify this and seek strategies and changes in his behaviour to prevent relapse are integral to recovery.

A lesser amount has been written on medical management, partly because of the lack of training referred to above, and partly because of a prejudice, I believe, that chemical abuse is someone else's problem. Nonetheless, there is a volume of work on the toxicology of alcoholism over the years and much recent work on harm minimisation through methadone programmes in opiate abuse.

But, so far as I am aware, there is no publication directly concerned with the short term, specialised, medical assistance of withdrawal from physical chemical dependency. I know this because I was almost accidentally (I now call it serendipity) asked to take over this role at Clouds in 1996, and I had absolutely no references to turn to. There must be many of us working in isolation around the world in various treatment centres, essentially reinventing the wheel in each location. The purpose of this reference therefore is to pass on what I have learnt from treating over a thousand patients. I continue to learn new things every day and I very much hope that a dialogue will ensue with others involved in this work so that we can share our knowledge and experiences.

Definitions

All patients that abuse chemicals will at an early stage attempt to validate their habit by denying that they have a problem, and by challenging the definition of the problem itself. I am sorry if it seems pedantic to spend time on defining exactly what or who this book concerns, but a brief semantic discussion is necessary, if only to avoid confusion.

Recreational drug use has been integral to social intercourse for as long as civilisation has been recorded. There is archaeological evidence of ritual chemical consumption among the ancient Egyptians, Chinese and Aztecs. Alcohol has been consumed in 'Public' houses for centuries, is used to augment celebrations between friends and allies, and is nearly always offered to visitors to one's home. North American Indians would pass the 'Peace Pipe' among their peers, in the same way that we see people passing a pack of cigarettes among their co-workers in the factory canteen. Sharing pleasurable (and sad) experiences is part of the social human condition, and sharing chemical experiences is no exception.

I tried to commence this book by using the expression 'chemical abuse'. That is fairly close, I think, to what should be concerning us. But, at the risk of sounding pious, it could be considered that any use of chemicals for other than medicinal purposes is abuse, and we all know that does not have to be the case.

In the case of alcohol the WHO and other health references state that there are 'safe limits', indeed, that small amounts are actually beneficial to health. That these limits are subject to wide individual variation is manifestly obvious as we all know of subjects who have lived to impressive ages despite heavy alcohol consumption. Similarly, there are some whose behaviour and bodies are damaged by relatively small amounts of alcohol consumed without apparent evidence of dependency. The term 'alcoholic' I presume means someone who suffers from physical withdrawal symptoms if his steady and heavy consumption is withdrawn. Therefore, I have always tried to avoid this term because it is too easy to disqualify from, the received assumption is that one has to be an alcoholic to be harmed by alcohol.

What we are concerned with here is **harm**. Where the use (or abuse) of any chemical results in harm to a person's body, mind, or the social microcosm in which he or she interacts, and specifically where that harm is deepening because of the loss of ability to control his or her use is what concerns us.

There are many who dip in and out of 'recreational' substance use. The 'social' drinker, the party goer who uses cocaine now and again. This does happen, I am not defending it, nor am I making any political comment. There are thousands of recreational drug users who do not develop significant harm from their irregular use, that is a fact. But there are some chemical users for whom the substance offers more than just an occasional pleasurable experience. We shall see that this relationship between chemical abuse and physical, psychological and social harm is a two way process. Very often, if not invariably, it is social, psychological or physical factors that create the valency for the chemical abuse. Alcohol is a powerful tranquilliser, it eases anxiety as opiates ease emotional pain. The emotionally damaged individual keeps revisiting the comfort of intoxication, but tolerance develops, doses need to be repeated more frequently, behaviour degrades and so the chemical abuse then progresses on to aggravate and inflame the pre-morbid condition.

Introduction

Euphemisms such as 'problem drinking' or 'misuse' are inadequate and confusing. In attempting to define our patient group perhaps it would be as well to take a few minutes to go back to first principles: the very need for treatment implies that to leave a condition untreated would lead to harm. In turn the word 'harm' in this context, means a continuing damage to the health of the patient's body and/or intellect and personality, and/or the social microcosm in which he exists, ie. his relationships with his family, partner, work and surrounding society. In examining the premorbid state of the patient it will be found almost invariably that a range of damage to one or more of these three dimensions already existed and indeed contributed directly to the substance abuse, so this process of harm works two-ways (*Tables 1 and 2*).

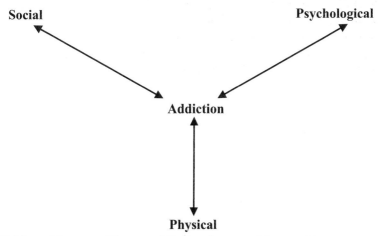

Table 1: Vectors of harm; addiction is caused by, and in turn causes damage to, the three dimensions of health

Table 2

Alcohol		Physical	Mental	Social
	CNS:	fits	Depression	isolation
		peripheral neuropathy	Psychosis	loss of self-respect
	Metabolics:	diabetes	Dementia	breakdown of relationships
		obesity	Amnesia	unemployment
		hyperlipidaemia	Insomnia	crime
		impotence	Anxiety	victimisation
	GI:	portal hypertension	Panic attacks	violence
		cirrhosis	DTS	divorce
		liver failure		loss of children
		liver cancer		abuse cycle
		gastritis/ulceration		exploitation
		pancreatitis		poverty
		malnutrition		road accidents
		aspiration pneumonia		hopelessness
		hypothermia		ghettoisation

	Physical	Psychological	Social
Opiates (from injecting):	sepsis	anhedonia	stigma
	DVT	loss of libido	loss
	gangrene	depression	rejection
	amputation	anxiety	underclass
	endocarditis	insomnia	prejudice
	HIV		uninsurable
	HCB, HBV		self-neglect
(other)	chronic bronchitis		self-hate
	malnutrition		self-harm
	accidental overdose		loss of education
	dental caries		perversion
Stimulants	Destruction of nasal mucosa		
	Cardiac: stress	anxiety	
	arrythmias	insomnia	
	papillary muscle rupture	depression	
	Skin changes (injecting harm as avove)		
	Dehydration		

Reproduced from a lecture given to patients in primary treatment. The categories on each axis were provided by the doctor and 30 patients in treatment filled in the grid, describing their own experiences of harm.

So far as substance abuse is concerned this harm is self-inflicted, yet the patient continues to carry out the activity that is causing the harm, which therefore implies a lack of control. It is true that often the patient does not recognise the harm, or blames others, or does not believe that he is harming himself. But this ignorance is usually short lived in the early stages of the problem behaviour. Before long logic dictates a causal relationship between the substance abuse and the harm being experienced, although this insight is frequently if not usually subverted by denial and diminishing consciousness through intoxication.

So for the purposes of this booklet I shall confine myself to those patients whose use of chemicals is harming one or more of these three elements of their health. It is a fairly pointless semantic argument to dwell on whether or not a patient is 'addicted' either physically or mentally. Suffice it to say that if a patient's abuse of mind affecting che
micals is harming himself or others around him, if he accepts that this is the case but recognises that he needs help because of his inability to control his use, then he needs treatment, whatever we choose to call him or his condition.

The definition of the patient group is an obvious one, and I do not anticipate much dispute from the above. However, there will be a variety of attitudes from professionals about how such patients should be helped and this is, to a large extent, a philosophical choice. I subscribe to the abstinence philosophy. I believe that the capacity to control consumption of mind affecting chemicals is like a ratchet, it only goes one way. For practical purposes, once control is lost it is never regained for long. Furthermore, once control is lost to one mind affecting chemical, the individual will be at very considerable risk of losing control if exposed to others. In other words, this patient group needs to recognise that treatment is aimed at a lifelong commitment to abstinence from **all** mind affecting substances. This booklet confines itself to these patients and their primary treatment:

that is the management of their medically assisted withdrawal from excessive uncontrolled use of mind affecting chemicals, with a view to a life without any such chemicals again.

After all, we aren't talking about vitamins here: heroin, alcohol, amphetamine, cocaine etc are all killers. They kill relationships, they kill minds and they kill people. Chemical abuse is by all criteria a terminal condition, yet it is the only terminal condition I know where the health professional can help the patient to usually arrest, and often reverse the process. This booklet is aimed at the medical aspect of this process but alone it will not succeed. Well-designed and effective primary treatment must address the patient's premorbid state, his personality and the way he has been moulded by his life's experiences. He must be helped to gain some insights, into his own behaviour and how this behaviour affects those around him. And, of course, he needs to learn strategies to help him change that behaviour where it risks relapse in the future.

Seeing patients years later into their abstinent 'recovery' looking healthy and happy is a remarkable and uplifting experience. Indeed, primary treatment for substance abuse is rather akin to midwifery: it is a very painful process but gives rise to new life, and is as rewarding for the caring professional as it gets.

Residential treatment

At the risk of stating the obvious, the point of treating chemical abuse is to minimise harm. There are measures that deliver large scale and very worthwhile reduction in harm without depending on abstinence; for instance, in an area where heroin misuse is widepread, the setting up of an agency to supply sterile hypodermic equipment alongside the judicious prescribing of methadone maintenance regimen has been demonstrated to be very significant in reducing crime, the spread of blood born viruses and other harm collateral to drug misuse.

In a 'herd' sense, such agencies are most beneficial to the population. However, on an individual patient basis, methadone maintenance, or other measures that go no further than containing the problem are not enough. In a population of chemical misusers there will be a substantial number at any one time who will want to escape from chronic chemical use and return to a life with an appropriate range of feelings. For these individuals who state that abstinence is their goal, how should this be achieved?

We know the answer to this question: well-designed residential treatment that combines detoxification with psychotherapy in a protected and nurturing environment has been repeatedly shown to have the most lasting benefit of any treatment model. Well-designed and skillful treatment comes at a premium cost; a six week period of primary residential treatment may cost from £4000 upwards. On the other hand, community based treatment costs a fraction of this sum and in a world where budgets are being constantly squeezed, the pressure will always be to offer detoxification and some sort of psychotherapy on an outpatient basis. It is my firm belief that commuity based treatment, although it may be successful for a number of patients, is beguiling. Every failed treatment sets the patient up as a failure and in so doing, makes future treatment more difficult. Well-designed residential treatment costs about the same as a knee replacement, a month of chemotherapy or a month of AIDS anti-viral therapy, with a similar outcome of success.

The success of residential treatment can be ascribed to a number of factors: clearly, removal from the using environment is essential, preferably to a treatment centre some distance away. To attempt to treat a patient who is still living within the home and environs where the cues to use are strongest invites relapse and failure. Similarly, removal of the patient from the home may give the family an opportunity for relief and support.

The intensive support that the patients and staff give to the individual, free of distractions, are also vital. Primary treatment is a most stressful time and this patient group has always responded to increasing stress by increasing use of mind affecting chemicals. In taking these chemicals away the patient has been denuded of his defence and he must have as much safety and support as possible. The cloistered life of the residential treatment centre offers this.

Finally, many of these patients are in a very frail state, and detoxification is itself a physically stressful and medically intensive situation. The residential treatment centre, with its expert medical staff available 24 hours a day, is the appropriate setting for these patients to start their recovery, to be detoxified, and to have their coexisting diseases appropriately addressed.

I am not suggesting that community detoxification has no place whatsoever. Where addiction is moderate, or perhaps the result of a reaction to a single crisis, it may well be worth attempting, indeed it may be a test of the severity of the problem. However, I am firmly of the opinion that if a patient presents us with the golden opportunity of seeking assistance toward abstinence, that evidence is overwhelmingly in favour of giving him the best opportunity to achieve this, through a well-designed residential programme. This book, therefore, is directed at medical personnel in residential treatment centres and advocates regimen that work in that context. Certain regimen, for instance the clonidine regime for detoxification from opiates, are wholly unsuitable for community use. Information is available elsewhere for those workers who wish to attempt detoxification in the community. However, at the risk of repeating myself this avenue should be selected only for what few merits it has, not its cheapness. It remains my firm belief that our patients have their best chance for lasting recovery through residential treatment, and further, that failure of community treatment invites the possibility of prejudicing successful treatment in the future.

Clouds House

Clouds is one of the United Kingdom's longest established and most respected residential treatment centres for the detoxification and primary treatment of those whose lives have been harmed by chemical abuse. It also has an academic tradition: in conjunction with the University of London it is the only UK treatment centre which offers a diploma course in training addiction counsellors, and is constantly engaged in a wide range of research.

Clouds offers a six week residential primary treatment as well as outpatient counselling services, education and family programmes. It accepts publicly funded and private patients from all over the United Kingdom and the World.

A range of educational materials, outcome analyses and other information is available from:

>Clouds House
>East Knoyle
>Salisbury
>Wiltshire
>SP3 6BE

Treatment philosophy, doctors as dealers, dual diagnosis

The medical service in residential primary treatment has four functions:

- to look at the applications of those seeking treatment and judge whether the individual is physically fit and prepared for the rigors of withdrawal and the daily activities in our community
- to attend to all the usual first aid, infections and other primary care problems that any group of people are affected with from time to time
- to attend to those physical conditions that are specific to this particular patient group
- to assist in the safe withdrawal from the substances that they have been abusing; a sometimes perilous but always difficult period, familiarly known as 'detox'.

This book is aimed at addressing these latter two aspects of medical care: so far as physical health issues particular to these patients is concerned, I shall not attempt to make an exhaustive treatise, there are far better medical texts already written that can be referred to in association with this book. But I will deal with those conditions that are important either because of their common incidence or because of their severity. I shall draw on my own experiences and how I have dealt with them.

Similarly the 'detoxification' schedules have been derived empirically from large patient numbers. They work for us, but I am well aware that there are many other workers in other centres who have their own various preferences. I would not advocate some of the methods that work for us in very different settings: as already stated, the clonidine protocol for opiate withdrawal I would judge to be wholly unsuitable for an outpatient in the community for reasons which will be explained later.

Our treatments are based on a number of philosophical tenets and practical considerations that may be particular to us, but I commend them to you if only because they work for many patients that have been through Clouds House.

The philosophical considerations are these: asking for help to become abstinent is a very brave undertaking, it is very difficult and indeed painful. Often our patients are at a very low ebb, their lives are in chaos, they have lost a great deal and feel full of shame. Undertaking primary treatment may be the first worthwhile thing that they have done in a very long time, and because it is so difficult it is an achievement which they can take justifiable pride in, in the future. That pride and sense of achievement are reinforcing forces to the survival of their recovery. Accordingly, for the medical team to take the whole process over and make it easy and painless devalues the patient's achievement. I do not take the puritanical view that if it doesn't hurt or taste horrible it won't work, but equally I do believe that our task is first and foremost to make the process safe, and secondary to that, to make it more bearable.

Having said that, patients' tolerances, motivations and situations generally vary, but to accomodate these variations by treating them individually invites exploitation. Many patients, either through fear, poor motivation or mischief will use the apparent 'extra' treatment of another patient as a reason to have their own treatment enhanced, and this is a very difficult argument to oppose. Unless there are clear, evident and medically compelling reasons to vary I would urge prescriptive and uniform regimen for all patient groups, ie. treat all opiate using patients with the same regimen, and all alcohol detoxification with the same uniform standards. I also feel it is imperative to remove 'as required' medications entirely unless they have no capacity to be abused. Accordingly hypnotics, sedatives of any kind, or codeine based pain killers should never be offered or given to the patient on demand.

The rewards of this policy are three-fold (*Table 3*). Firstly, the medical staff's job will be made far easier by the minimisation of patients attempting to manipulate their treatment if they know that it is pointless to try. Secondly, the patient's pattern of behaviour in the past has always been to go to the off-licence, or dealer and obtain a supply of 'medication' when he feels in need and this behaviour is continuing into treatment. In asking for treatment he has accepted that he needs help to control his abuse of psychoactive chemicals and we are therefore helping him by so refusing. Finally, the psychotherapeutic aspect of primary treatment demands that the patient expresses appropriate feelings; his historical behaviour has always been to wash unpleasant feelings away in a chemical haze, and if this continues into his psychotherapy the opportunity to experience appropriate feelings and learn how to deal with them will have been lost. It is the task of the medical arm of the treatment team to support their psychotherapy colleagues by removing psychoactive treatments as soon as it is safe to do so. The watchwords are clarity, consistency and fairness.

Table 3: Rigid protocols offer:
* minimisation of the potential for manipulation by the patient
* reinforcement and support for the patient's expressed intentions by **not** answering the feeling of need for intoxication
* the briefest route to abstinence from all mind affecting chemicals facilitiates the psychotherapeutic arm of treatment.

A real difficulty arises when the patient has been prescribed psycho-active medication by his doctors in the community. If a psychoactive drug has been authorised by a trusted health professional, often making the patient feel better, a number of difficult issues arise:

- the patient will be exposed to a conflict of advice which may undermine his confidence in our treatment
- the patient may be returned to that same doctor's care after primary treatment and hence be advised a return to the same treatment
- the drug may actually be necessary.

This last statement may sound obvious, but should be explained; doctors are caring people, they want to make their patients feel better. They often have long term, close, even collusive relationships with their patients where they are reluctant to withhold a treatment that the patient wants in case refusal may jeopardise that long term relationship (we only have to consider the vast over prescribing of antibiotics to see that). Doctors often know that their treatment is not strictly necessary but make a judgement that is 'expedient'. In so doing, short term gain is often bought at the cost of long term pain.

We are all familiar with the consequences of the over zealous prescribing of benzodiazepines in the 1960s. Prior to the introduction of Valium and its descendants, doctors had some pretty unpleasant drugs to use as sedatives, notably barbiturates which were known to be very addictive and were responsible for many hundreds of deaths annually from intentional (and unintentional) overdose. The new benzodiazepines were hailed as being extremely effective and comforting to patients, safe in overdose (which they certainly are) and non addictive (which they certainly are not). We now live with the consequence of a generation of people brought up then (and a number since) who are habituated to tranquillisers and sleeping pills. But if that is an obvious and gross example of the doctors iatrogenic harm through care, there are other more subtle examples, especially with antidepressants.

Modern antidepressants are fairly safe, relatively non-habituating and effective. A doctor knows that an unhappy patient may feel better on an antidepressant even though he knows that the vast majority of his patients become depressed as a reaction to adverse life events. When a person becomes depressed reactively, it may be entirely appropriate to be so as, for instance, when bereaved. If that reaction is inappropriately prolonged or severe there may be complex psychological reasons why this is so, which need to be addressed. Although it is likely that these new drugs are not physically harmful, and frequently do not have a withdrawal syndrome, nonetheless they are being prescibed inappropriately in such situations as they disable the patient from reacting appropriately and inhibit emotions from responding naturally. Furthermore, prescribing 'treatment' fosters the belief that is increasingly prevalent in modern society that negative feeling is a disease and should be medicated away, and in the specific case of the substance abuser this reinforces his own harmful behaviour. A psychotherapeutic approach may be more time consuming, difficult and expensive even, but it will empower the patient to respond to life's 'slings and arrows' more appropriately in the future. The expedient use of antidepressants disempowers the patient's own resources.

I do not want to oversimplify this situation as it is a complex one; there are indeed some patients who despite having stable and fulfilling relationships, and other rewards in life, still go through phases of being profoundly depressed. There is often a family history of depression, sometimes with psychotic features and for these individuals there may well be a primary neurochemical imbalance that would be appropriately treated with antidepressants. Similarly, there are other psychiatric illnesses that may be caused by substance abuse, or may have predated the abuse and so contributed to it. Such patients may function more happily and appropriately with psychoactive medication, indeed, may revert to being very disturbed and mentally ill if the medication is removed. This is a very difficult area: our primary concern is clearly to address the harmful behaviour of illicit substance or excessive alcohol abuse and to that extent we should not jeopardise the patient's treatment by interfering inappropriately in necessary psychoactive medication.

Equally, such medication may interfere with the patient's ability to respond appropriately to the psychotherapeutic approach, by chemically modulating appropriate emotional responses and behaviour. There is no prescriptive answer here. Each patient's diagnosis and treatment has to be very carefully assessed by skilled practitioners familiar with mental illness and with our therapeutic approach, and judgement must be made as to whether we should attempt primary treatment, or whether it should be attempted elsewhere by those with an approach more suited to that individual. We owe it to the patient to refuse him treatment if we do not think that abstinence based treatment is appropriate at this stage. To set him up for likely failure is not only wanton but also undermines his success with subsequent treatment attempts elsewhere.

Alcohol — physical harm and withdrawal syndrome

Table 4: The physical effects of alcohol	
Nutritional state:	obesity muscle atrophy vitamin deficiency hypoproteinaemia predisposition to infection

Liver disease:	fatty degeneration
	alcoholic hepatitis
	cirrhosis: portal hypertension
	                   oesophageal varices
	                   ascites
	hepatic failure
	hepatoma (primary liver cancer)

other gastrointestinal:	gastritis peptic ulceration pancreatitis
The nervous system:	peripheral neuropathy The Wernicke-Korsakoff syndrome cerebellar ataxia amblyopia epileptiform seizures
Metabolic:	diabetes hyperlipidaemia impotence
Cardiovascular:	hypertension cardiomyopathy ischaemic heart disease

There can be few parts of the body that are unaffected by chronic excess of alcohol although we tend to dwell on the liver and nervous system because these are most commonly and severely affected. Diabetes, with all its attendant complications, heart disease, gastritis, ulceration, pancreatitis, impotence, even psoriasis and Dupuytrens palmar contracture are all contributed to and sometimes exclusively caused by alcoholism. Medical textbooks will provide the interested reader with exhaustive accounts of the physical harm to the body from alcohol, I shall confine myself here to those severe or frequently encountered problems which merit our attention in primary treatment.

Nutrition

As with most expensive and compelling habits, chronic heavy drinkers usually neglect their diet. This is a particular problem for the alcohol abuser who will malabsorb vitamins and has impaired liver function and protein synthesis. The body will preferentially burn ethanol as a calorific source over fat so the cumulative affect of these factors in the chronic heavy drinker is frequently a clinical picture of an obese patient with low muscle bulk, low stamina and a susceptibility to infections. Males may demonstrate gynaecomastia and suffer from impotence.

Liver disease

Chronic heavy alcohol consumption leads to a syndrome of liver damage which commences with fatty degeneration, proceeding to alcoholic hepatitis, cirrhosis, liver failure and sometimes hepatoma (primary liver cancer). Once cirrhotic, the clinical picture may be complicated by portal hypertension, which may present for the first time with a torrential and often fatal bleed from oesophageal varices. Other features of portal hypertension are the rare so-called 'Caput

Medusa' sign of engorged veins around the umbilicus, and severe haemorrhoids. Degrees of hepatomegaly vary from modest to immense, associated with a variable amount of ascites. Frank jaundice is a poor prognostic indicator, and may deepen during the stress of detoxification. Prognosticating in alcoholic liver damage is very imprecise, the liver is an enormously forgiving organ and if abstinence is maintained, demonstrates a very considerable power to recover sufficiently for the body's future demands. Blood testing of liver function is singularly unhelpful during primary treatment, though often requested by the anxious patient. The profile so soon after admission will almost always look terrible with grossly elevated GGT levels, and if it isn't, may encourage the patient to feel that he can return to drinking with impunity. If abstinence is maintained then LFT estimation after six months or so should be more valid, with persistent abnormality indicating chronic irreversible damage, though again, there is little more that can be done apart from liver transplantation.

Central nervous system (CNS) disease

The alcohol abuser invariably develops his habit through using ethanol for its tranquillising properties. It is a very effective short acting tranquilliser, but it depresses not only the higher intellect's anxiety but the entire nervous system's functions. The persistent dampening down of nervous stimulation leads to an insidious lowering of excitation thresholds.

The drinker will recognise this over the course of time by his anxiety levels worsening, panic attacks, insomnia, involuntary shaking, delirium tremens (hallucinations, usually frightening visual images of crawling insects etc) and epileptiform seizures.

Apart from the direct effect of alcohol, there is further more substantial damage to neural tissue from induced vitamin B deficiency. The central nervous sytem (CNS) is highly dependent on

B vitamins, which become deficient in the chronic heavy drinker because of reduced absorption, poor diet and increased demand. This can lead to glove and stocking parasthesae, similar to the picture of subacute combined degeneration of the cord known as alcoholic peripheral neuropathy, cerebellar ataxia, the Wernicke-Korsakoff syndrome and rarely, total amblyopia.

The B vitamin most implicated in causing CNS harm through deficiency is thiamine, though pyridoxine, riboflavine and niacin are also involved. In acute withdrawals the sudden increase in metabolic demand may totally deplete the paltry reserves of thiamine, leading to a sudden clouding of consciousness, opthalmoplegia and ataxia, a syndrome known as Wernicke's encephalopathy. This is often fatal, and if survived, 25% go on to a permanent state of dementia and ataxia known as Korsakoff's psychosis. The Wernicke-Korsakoff syndrome (WKS) is of vital importance to the medical team involved in alcohol detoxification, and all staff should be intimately aware of its signs and symptoms because of its very serious consequences and its near total avoidability. The condition is uncommon but even so, more common than is widely thought (Cook and Thomson, 1997). Predicting who is likely to be affected is difficult but obviously those malnourished, with chronic heavy consumption and other signs of CNS or liver disease will be at greatest risk. If there is **any** significant concern that the patient may be at risk, he must be given high potency vitamin B complex quickly and in large dosage **parenterally** as the oral route is rendered almost totally useless because of compromised absorption.

Skin

Skin changes in alcoholics are not often written about in medical texts and although not particularly significant are quite common in my experience and worthy of mention. Psoriasis is an unusual but sometimes severe event, but what is much more common is an often widespread dermatitis. This can affect the face and scalp, the trunk, arms and legs in decreasing order of frequency. It has the typical appearance of an acute eczema, sometimes with psoriatic features. Often during and after detoxification patients will complain of widespread itching and desquamation even if their dermatitis was not apparent on admission. It is probably best treated with simple emollients but steroid creams may be needed in severe cases.

Telangectasia, specifically the so-called 'spider' naevi are seen in more significant liver disease and may be occasional or numerous and florid. Jaundice is a sign of cirrhosis, caused by both compromised hepatic function and a degree of cirrhotic intra hepatic biliary obstruction, it is a poor prognostic indicator. It may also be a sign of hepatoma.

Acne, usually acne rosacea, rhinophyma and other skin infections are frequently seen, and improve rapidly once abstinence and renutrition take place. Dupuytrens palmar contracture is seen infrequently and may need surgical fasciotomy at some future date.

Other physical changes

Many long term alcohol abusers are hypertensive, and may also suffer from dyspeptic problems. It is remarkable how quickly both of these conditions may settle, frequently completely, on no treatment other than alcohol withdrawal.

Diabetes is usually caused by a combination of pancreatic damage to insulin production and increased demand through the high calorific content of the volume of alcohol consumption. A variable response is seen in the diabetic who becomes abstinent; most will see an improvement in their blood sugars, indeed the insulin controlled patient will have to be wary of hypoglycaemia and it is prudent to put the patient on a sliding scale of insulin according to his blood sugar levels, until stability is regained.

It is fair to say that this patient group neglects its health badly and the early stages of medically assisted withdrawal are a golden opportunity to address many outstanding health problems.

Alcohol — treatment principles and aims

As has already been stated, the aims for the medical team in treating substance abusing patients is twofold, namely:

● to assist the patient to abstinence safely and quickly

● to treat any illness consequential to their substance abuse.

A history of the patient's drinking pattern will assist the physician in forming a picture of what may be expected on withdrawal. I should emphasise that the medical team in a treatment centre for addiction should always be prepared for any unforeseen eventuality, as we are dealing with a health situation that is in many cases very difficult to predict. Furthermore, patients' histories are frequently unreliable; our patient group almost always come from a background of years of deception both in dealing with others and themselves. Although they are seeking to change their behaviour by entering treatment, dishonesty is almost second nature to this population and the prudent physician would be well advised to remain open-minded when listening to the history that they give.

Nonetheless, a history is needed: alcohol abusers are a diverse group, and their medical needs in treatment are similarly heterogenous. Clearly the 'bingeing' alcohol abuser who may go for days or weeks on a recurring basis with no alcohol consumption at all is well used to abrupt cessation, he does it all the time at home. His needs from the medical team will be quite distinct from those of the daily drinker with a history of withdrawal seizures, malnutrition and so forth.

As soon as possible after admission the physician must see and examine the patient, and prescribe the appropriate medication to assist in the safe withdrawal from alcohol (see *Table 5*).

If as happens frequently, the patient arrives heavily intoxicated, some of the examination may have to be postponed until the patient becomes sober but no longer than is absolutely neccessary.

General considerations

The patient needs close monitoring in the first 24–48 hours of treatment for signs of severe CNS excitation and/or Wernicke's encephalopathy. Sedative medication is seldom needed after five to seven days, but may be needed liberally at first. Thereafter, the patient will be anxious, insomniac and frail, but little if any medication is needed after ten days or so. From then on, priority is given to renourishing the patient and rehabilitating what are usually extremely unfit people.

Patients must have their pulse, blood pressure and temperature checked four to six times in the first 24 hours, then less frequently as their condition stabilises and improves. Signs of CNS excitation, such as tachycardia, raised blood pressure, shaking, or the patient reporting flashing lights, spots in his vision etc, are all signs to administer further sedation. Blurred vision, clouding of consciousness, ataxia, lowering temperature may be signs of impending Wernicke's encephalopathy and merit increasing parenteral vitamin B therapy.

Table 5: The physician's history and examination — alcohol

History	Significant past general medical history Prescribed medication (for any purpose) Allergies Other drug consumption, not prescribed
Drinking history	Duration of problem drinking Frequency of drinking, ie. daily or bingeing Typical amount Daily pattern: what time do they start drinking? (drinking early in the day is often found in patients who experience severe withdrawal symptoms, ie. retching, shaking and who need alcohol to become 'well' enough to get through the day) Last time that they went three consecutive days without a drink — what was it like? Any history of fitting, delirium tremens

Examination	A general examination as appropriate
	An examination specific to alcohol abusers:
	    evidence of recent head injury from falls, bruises, bumps should invoke a careful neurological assessment in case of insidious intracranial bleeding, ie. subdural haematoma
	General nutritional state
	Stigmata of diseases of chronic alcohol excess:
	    sclera, for signs of jaundice
	    hepatomegaly, splenomegaly
	    gynaecomastia
	    Dupuytrens contracture
	    caput medusa
	    ascites
	    spider naevi, telangectases
	    lower limb oedema
	    glove and stocking parasthesae
	    ataxia, Rombergism

Medication

Sedation

The principle of medically assisted alcohol withdrawal is to transfer the patient from alcohol to a safer sedative, then acclimatize the central nervous sytem to becoming drug free, by weaning off over a safe and short period. The most commonly used sedative drugs to achieve this are chlordiazepoxide, diazepam and chlormethiazole (Heminevrin). Personally, I do not favour Heminevrin. It is not as safe as the benzodiazepines, has some toxicity and is less predictable. Having said that, it is extremely powerful and I have used it in an intensive care situation in hospital by continuous intravenous infusion, where it is highly effective. I would not argue against its use by the physician who is experienced in its use in the residential setting, however I continue to be saddened by the number of well meaning practitioners who prescribe chlormethiazole in the unsupervised outpatient context. This drug is absolutely contraindicated with concurrent alcohol consumption and unless such a possibility can be excluded (ie. in residential treatment) it should never be prescribed. There continue to be fatalities from this cause each year, all of them avoidable.

Diazepam and chlordiazepoxide are both extremely effective in sedating the patient during alcohol withdrawal, both also have some anti-epileptic effect and have enormous latitudes of safety. I would not care to advocate one over the other, my prejudice is to favour chlordiazepoxide as I feel it has less 'reward' for the patient but there is, I confess, little science in this preference.

Control of seizures

A treatment unit has to accept the possibility of epileptic seizures among its patients at any time, indeed the patients must accept this

risk when coming off virtually all mind affecting chemicals, especially alcohol and benzodiazepines. The risk is maximal toward the end of sedative treatment, but is still a significant though diminishing risk for several days after discontinution. It might be considered desirable to minimise the risk of seizures by giving anti-convulsant medication routinely in all alcohol or benzodiazepine detoxes, until about ten days after completion. The argument against doing so would be that this is extra sedative medication that can make some patients very drowsy, has other side effects, is in the great majority of cases unnecessary and cannot guarantee that no seizures will ever occur. Who is treated with anti-convulsant drugs is therefore a matter of choice, a compromise of risk management. My preference is to give anti-convulsant medication to:

- all patients with a previous history of epileptic or withdrawal seizures
- all patients being detoxified from continuous benzodiazepine or barbiturate use of over ten years
- any other alcohol or benzodiazepine abusing patient who has had a heavy and continuous use, who after being counselled about the risk of seizures, wishes to minimise it.

Given the choice of modern anti-epileptic medication, I favour carbamazepine, though phenytoin is also effective. Barbiturates are clearly to be avoided for obvious reasons, valproate is a third choice but probably less effective in this field, and the newer drugs such as lamotrigine have yet to prove themselves in withdrawal seizures.

Vitamin B

Alcohol abusing patients become depleted in vitamin B complex for three reasons: their vitamin requirements are high, they tend to neglect their diet, and alcohol inhibits the gut's capacity to absorb vitamin B. The first tissue in the body to experience the harmful effects of vitamin B deficiency is neural tissue.

Chronic vitamin B deficiency may cause the insidious progression of peripheral neuropathy (glove and stocking parasthesae), impotence, and rarely sudden painless ambylopia, which may be bilateral and permanent. However, it is the sudden depletion of vitamin B in alcohol withdrawal that concerns us most.

Alcohol withdrawal is metabolically demanding and small vitamin B stores can become abruptly depleted. This may lead to acute changes in the brain, with symptoms of opthalmoplegia, ataxia and clouding of consciousness, the syndrome of Wernicke's encephalopathy (see *page 10*). The Wernicke-Korsakov syndrome is tragic and entirely preventable with adequate vitamin replacement. The vitamins implicated, usually thiamine, but also pyridoxine, riboflavine and niacin, must be administered parenterally if WKS is seriously considered a risk. Oral administration is **never** adequate owing to poor absorbtion in the alcoholic gut. The preparation that is used in the UK is Pabrinex. It's forebear, Parenterovite, fell from favour because of reports of anaphylactic reactions. Pabrinex has been widely used over the past decade or so, and given intramuscularly causes anaphylaxis in 1 in 5,000,000 doses. There should be little if any caution therefore in prescribing it to the alcohol abuser who comes into treatment.

The injections are quite painful and WKS may only affect 2% or so of chronic alcohol abusers in withdrawal so some judgement may be possible as to who should receive it: bingeing alcohol abusers with good diets are probably at small risk, but the malnourished and overtly liver damaged patient should always receive parenteral vitamins. The physician risks little in giving Pabrinex, but potentially much in withholding it.

Table 6: Medication used in alcohol detoxification	
Sedation	chlordiazepoxide or diazepam
Control of seizures	carbamazepine or phenytoin
Parenteral B vitamins	

Reference

Cook CH, Thomson AD (1997) B-complex vitamins in the prophylaxis and treatment of Wernicke-Korsakoff syndrome. *Br J Hosp Med* **57**(9): 461–465

The sedatives — benzodiazepine and barbiturate abuse, physical harm and withdrawal syndromes

This is perhaps an opportune point to discuss dependency to pharmaceutical sedatives. These drugs are usually abused by the same type of patient who abuses alcohol, indeed abuse of the two commonly co-exist in the same patient. They work on a similar place in the brain, and cause very similar withdrawal states. The most important difference is that most pharmaceutical sedatives (notably excluding meprobamate and chloral derivatives) are not toxic to the liver, nor do they degrade neural tissue in the same irreversible way as alcohol does. Although they do not cause much in the way of physical harm, they induce tolerance and dependency, and provoke a most unpleasant and lengthy period of withdrawal symptoms, particularly of anxiety and panic attacks, but also parasthesae and epileptiform seizures. The initial rush of enthusiasm to change patients from barbiturates to benzodiazepines (BZDs) in the 1960s under the mistaken belief that they were non toxic and non addictive has left a legacy of many thousands of people with serious benzodiazepine dependency. We are grateful that we no longer see the many thousands of both accidental and deliberate self-poisonings from barbiturates, but that should now be tempered by cautious and prudent use of the benzodiazepines, ever wary of their very considerable potential for addiction.

The degree and duration of withdrawal symptoms are very variable between patients, being more severe with length of abuse, amount of drug used and type of drug used, lorazepam having distinctly the worst withdrawal syndrome of all the benzodiazepines.

Uniquely (almost) among chemicals of abuse and addiction, pharmaceutical sedative dependency may arise from over zealous or injudicious prescribing by the medical profession. This introduces a particular difficulty in treatment, in that the administration has been sanctioned, or validated, by doctors themselves. As the withdrawal process unearths uncomfortable and sometimes terrifying anxiety attacks, the patient will very reasonably question whether he should be in treatment at all: after all, why should one doctor do the exact opposite of another? Furthermore, after completion of treatment the patient will usually be returned to the same well-intentioned practitioner who has been collusive in the patient's addiction. The medical team therefore has a difficult role of diplomatic re-education of both patient and doctor to ensure a lasting recovery.

The medical assistance of BZD withdrawal, and (rarely these days) barbiturate withdrawal, is identical to that of alcohol withdrawal, with the following notable exceptions:

- patients will rarely have liver or lasting neural damage and will generally be much more physically fit than those abusing alcohol
- there is no risk of WKS and no need for vitamin administration
- the risk of epileptiform seizures is greater
- the duration of anxiety attacks, insomnia and agitation will be much longer, the risk of acute psychotic disturbance greater and the sedative weaning process also much lengthier, complicated by severe headaches, visual disturbances and insomnia.

Accordingly, carbamazepine will be needed frequently, and the daily use of sedatives converted into an equivalent dose of diazepam to be split into two to four doses per day (*Table 7*) and reduced over a much longer period than with alcohol. Unless under very exceptional circumstances, I believe that chronicity of even decades of continuous benzodiazepine use can be weaned off over three weeks or so, rarely longer. This process is always distressing and patients may be left with unresolved anxiety and insomnia many months or even years later. But the weaning can be done **safely** in three weeks or so.

Table 7: Potency of benzodiazepines	
The approximate relative potency of benzodiazepines to diazepam 10 mg are as follows:	
chlordiazepoxide	30 mg
diazepam	10 mg
flunitrazepam	1 mg
flurazepam	30 mg
nitrazepam	10 mg
loprazolam	2 mg
lorazepam	1 mg
lormetazepam	2 mg
nitrazepam	10 mg
oxazepam	30 mg
temazepam	20 mg
triazolam	0.75 mg

The opiates — physical harm, withdrawal syndromes and medical management

Opiate addiction is prevalent and growing worldwide, it is as important numerically in primary treatment centres as alcohol addiction. Casual use of opiates is becoming more common and because of its addictive properties, tolerance and dependency frequently follow.

The patient is often exposed to the heroin first by smoking it rolled up with tobacco in the same way as hashish, in a 'joint'. A better 'hit' is obtained by smoking the drug unadulterated by heating it from below on a piece of aluminium foil, and inhaling the fumes through a tube, a process known as 'chasing (the dragon)'. Intravenous injection is subsequently sought as a way of enhancing the hit, and using the drug more efficiently.

Heroin induces euphoria and sedation and, of course, analgesia. For a typical opiate user a dose lasts two to three hours before cravings set in, characterised physically by shivering and skin crawling sensations, with epiphora and rhinorrhoea that become progressively more intense. Later painful muscle spasms develop, often in the loins and the patient becomes extremely agitated. The heroin addict therefore needs to repeat his dose three or four times daily. When unemployed this is a costly business and the addict may resort to criminal activities to sustain the habit. Theft, supply of drugs and prostitution are commonplace, enhancing the patient's feelings of worthlessness and self-disgust, factors that further contribute to heroin use.

There are considerable health risks particularly to the injecting drug user, and many authorities have seized on prescription of heroin substitutes as a means of harm minimisation; in the UK the favoured drug of replacement is methadone, in France codeine or buprenorphine, in Switzerland even pharmaceutical heroin itself. Stabilisation on these drugs gives the patient a way out of criminal activity, and a way out of exposing himself to the risks of self-injection, particularly shared self-injection (see below).

Many studies have shown that this policy of harm minimisation is extremely effective at reducing harm and criminal activity. But this policy is not without its own problems. For instance, the liberal availability of methadone in the UK has washed a lot of the drug onto the black market where some individuals (notably children) are unused to its high potency, and the number of fatalities each year from accidental overdosage is double that of heroin itself. Even with a regular prescription for substitution medicine, most addicts continue to use heroin, albeit to a lesser degree, and there is evidence that methadone 'maintained' patients use increasing amounts of alcohol and benzodiazepines. Nonetheless, the policy of substitution or 'maintenance' therapy is a proven one and, on balance, does have some merit. However, it should be matched by a commitment to primary abstinence-directed treatment for the regular number of addicts each year who want to escape the dependency culture and become drug free. This is a political and health economic argument which, although an important debate, I shall not expand further upon as it is outside the remit of this small volume. In the author's view, methadone maintenance therapy in the UK has become a preoccupation to the exclusion of abstinence, and I feel that the balance needs to be redressed.

So far as primary treatment is concerned, it has been our policy to treat all opiate users in exactly the same prescriptive way, as will be described below. It must be said that heroin addiction is far easier to withdraw from than methadone addiction. Methadone withdrawal symptoms last longer and are more profound than those of heroin.

Consequential harm from opiate addiction

Table 8: Physical harm from opiates		
From the drug itself:	anorexia — poor nutritional state	
	anhedonia — lack of self-care	
From inorganic injection contaminants	phlebitis	
	vessel destruction:	ischaemia
		false aneurysm
		arteriovenous fistula
		gangrene
	peripheral oedema	
From organic (pathogen) injection contaminants	bacteria:	abcess formation locally and distant
		septicaemia
		subacute bacterial endocarditis
	viruses:	hepatitis C
		hepatitis B
		human immunodeficiency virus

Heroin itself is relatively harmless to the body. That may seem a rash and irresponsible statement, but it is true nonetheless. Codeine or pharmaceutical morphine or diamorphine (heroin) addiction is very well recognised in medicine, indeed it is often created by doctor's prescription. We know that these drugs produce little physical harm other than constipation, weight loss and anhedonia. However, great harm arises from the self-administration of opiates that have been contaminated by impurities and, far worse, pathogenic microbes.

Smoking

'Chasing' heroin is an age old method of administration yet there is comparatively little written in professional papers about its long term effects. Opium has been smoked in dens in the Far East, in Victorian England and elsewhere for many years. It is likely that if it were more harmful than tobacco we would know about it by now, so it is probable that its physical consequences are few. My own observations are that patients frequently have very unhealthy sounding chests with coarse bronchospasm which is often confused with asthma. Indeed, many patients arrive in treatment with asthma inhalers that have been prescibed by doctors who may have been unaware of their patient's drug habits. These chest sounds improve steadily in the first few weeks of abstinence.

Injecting, harm from inorganic impurities

Illicit heroin is manufactured by inexpert chemists and then diluted by being 'cut' with various impurities such as salt, sugar, talcum powder and various other substances, even brick dust. To make it go into solution so that it can be injected, the addict will mix his impure heroin with ascorbic acid, lemon juice etc and tap water, heat it up on a spoon, aspirate the result though a cigarette filter to take out the lumps and then inject it direct into his venous circulation. This introduces the potential for harm in a number of ways; firstly, inexpert autoinjection of a solution that contains many impurities leads to superficial thrombophlebitis and subsequent sclerosis of veins. As the veins of the arms are exhausted, the patient will move on to the veins of the feet and legs, the large veins in the groins and neck, and even the tiny venules in the penis, eyelid etc when through desperation, no other veins are found. Progressive loss of venous channels may lead to gross and disfiguring swelling of the limbs, but worse, missing the veins and hitting adjacent arteries, particularly in the groin and antecubital fossae, may sclerose the artery and lead to acute ischaemia of the limb, leading to contracture, or gangrene and amputation.

Injecting, harm from pathogenic microbes

There is no deliberate virus contamination of heroin supplies, but addicts tend to self-inject in groups and their ignorance of safe injection techniques together with desperation may invite the cross contamination of blood born virusses. In the past few years this risk must be known by virtually all intravenous drug abusers, and the ready availability of sterile syringes and needles from street agencies might lead one to suppose that this is now a redundant risk.

Sadly however, addicts continue to become infected by reusing hypodermic equipment that may be communal, and using cleaning or other techniques that they mistakenly believe to be safe.

The most significant viral infection is that of hepatitis C which is thought to be present in 40–100% of injecting drug abusers, depending on locality. The virus may survive ouside the body for months or years and is so infectious that a single injection with a well washed but shared needle may be enough to transmit the infection. Primary treatment health workers should obtain an intimate knowledge of hepatitis B and C from suitable textbooks, but hepatitis C is a very serious infection. It has only been identified for the past 20 years or so, previously it was clumsily known as 'non A, non B hepatitis'. It seems that the large majority of infected patients go on to develop chronic active hepatitis with consequent cirrhosis and eventual liver failure over a varying and unpredictable time span. It is likely that all infected patients are lifelong carriers of infection.

Of lesser significance, both numerically and in severity, is hepatitis B, which is also very infectious by sharing injecting equipment, but its lesser frequency probably reflects a need for a higher innoculation of virus particles for infection to occur, than hepatitis C. However, it is more infectious venereally than hepatitis C. Hepatitis B is usually a self-limiting episode but 25% of patients become chronic carriers of the infection, and a lesser number follow a course similar to that of hepatitis C.

The great *bête-noir* of viral blood infections is, of course, HIV. This infection is to be found among drug users not only because of its ready spread among those sharing intravenous equipment, but also because it is infectious venerally and prostitution (by definition with many partners) is a commonly used fundraising activity by female and male heroin addicts. Intravenous drug abuse is now the most common source of HIV infection in the UK and its infection rate remains pretty constant despite widespread health education over the past few years. It would be usual for most primary treatment centres to have at least one HIV infected patient in treatment at any one time and the medical team must therefore become acquainted with the health needs of this population. Modern antiviral therapies have considerably extended these patients' life expectancies, many looking to abstinence as a way of further enhancing their prognosis.

Finally, the lack of aseptic techniques may further lead to abscess formation along the course of veins and the introduction of pathogenic skin bacteria. This can develop into full blown septicaemia, collapse, renal failure and death, or may insidiously lead to bacterial endocarditis, brain abscess, osteomyelitis etc.

Treatment

The treatment goals remain the same for all patients with addiction: to achieve a safe and speedy transition to abstinence, and to treat any illness consequent to their substance abuse.

However unlike, for instance, alcohol withdrawal, there are few if any serious potential physical hazards in the withdrawal process, so the priority of achieving a safe withdrawal is not so acute. The main aim is to achieve as speedy a transition to being opiate free as is reasonable, bearing in mind that this can be an uncomfortable process. To repeat one of the aims of treatment that was given in the opening to this book, our task is to help the addict with his stated intention to become abstinent, not to completely take the task, and so achievement, away from him. This is an important point in treating opiate addiction: our task is to make the withdrawal process bearable, while at the same time being clear, consistent and fair.

In a treatment centre we will come across patients of different ages with a widely differing consumption of drugs. Intravenous preparations of methadone are being prescribed by some practitioners (usually privately) in quantities that I would find hard to justify. We may be asked at one moment to withdraw a patient from 250 mg of injected pharmaceutical methadone daily, and at another, one who smokes a '£10 bag of brown' three times a day. To treat them differently seems obvious, yet invites manipulation and the perception of inequality between peers in treatment together. To use the alcohol or sedative model of assisted withdrawal (above), it would be logical to prescribe an amount of methadone equal to the patient's use, then wean him off. This invites all the opiate abusing patients in the community to claim vast habits and to vie with the doctor for larger amounts of methadone because they had understated their previous use.

While in the grip of addiction, opiate abusers are particularly adept at manipulating and attempting to influence their treatment through deception or by whatever means they hope will succeed. They tend to exaggerate their consumption and maximise the severity of the withdrawal symptoms that they are experiencing in order to obtain as much drug therapy as possible. They should not be blamed for this, this is behaviour acquired through years of dealing with unsympathetic doctors and is often almost second nature. Besides which, opiate withdrawals are both painful and frightening and a wish to ease this discomfort has understandably been their habit every day for years. Clonidine (or lofexidine) has revolutionised my treatment of these patients in the residential setting (detailed below) in that it completely dispenses with inequalities by being applicable to all opiate addicts, regardless of their previous usage. Furthermore, with the protocol that I shall detail, all patients will be opiate free within 48 hours of entering treatment. In the residential setting, where we have our patients for a continuous period of several weeks, there is almost never any need to vary from the clonidine or lofexidine protocol.

It is also worth mentioning that these drugs are largely unknown to opiate abusers as they have no potential for abuse. It is advantageous if the regime to be employed can be explained and agreed ('contracted' if you will) prior to admission. This saves a great deal of argument when the patient is suddenly faced by the frightening prospect of imminent withdrawal, as soon as he arrives in treatment.

Treatment should take place as soon as possible after admission (*Table 9*).

Following history taking and examination, the detoxification process should be explained in detail to the patient. It should be clearly stated that the object is to make withdrawal bearable, not take all symptoms away — the patient must understand that withdrawal symptoms are inevitable, that he will feel uncomfortable, that he will have difficulty sleeping and, moreover, that the treatment regime will not be varied from under any circumstances. It should be emphasised in a supportive way that what is being prescribed is realistic and based on very extensive experience of many patients whose use has been the same or greater than his own.

Table 9: Physician's guide to history and examination of the opiate user

Past medical history of significant health problems:

* prescribed medication in the recent weeks prior to admission
* allergies
* a detailed list of the patient's current drug use from all sources. This may be difficult, as many drug abusers have irregular supplies and chaotic habits, but as clear a picture as possible is needed, routes of administration, and when last dosed
* alcohol history
* last menstrual period in females, possibility of pregnancy.

General examination, with emphasis on the following:

* an inspection of injection sites, with attention to evidence of abscesses
* thrombophlebitis, false femoral aneurysms, distal swelling
* heart sounds, signs of bronchospasm
* abdominal examination, with attention to loading of the descending colon from chronic constipation, and tenderness of the liver, hepatomegaly
* stigmata of HIV infection such as Kaposis sarcomata, fungal infections, unexplained weight loss
* mouth for candidiasis and dental caries.

I have used the combination therapy in *Table 10* to assist the withdrawal of hundreds of opiate addicted patients whose use has varied enormously, from over 300 mg of pharmaceutical morphine per day, or 250 mg of injected methadone a day, to a modest codeine habit. All patients are completely opiate-free after just 48 hours, and free of all mind affecting substances by the fifth day. The regime described is tolerated by virtually all patients although with variable degrees of discomfort, and is vital to the early introduction of the psycho-therapeutic activities.

Table 10: Drugs used in opiate detoxification
Clonidine or lofexidine — to ease opiate withdrawal symptoms
Methadone* in low dose to bridge the first 48 hours before full clonidine dose
Oxazepam for four nights
(* may be replaced with codeine or buprenorphine if this is the patient's drug of choice)

Methadone

Methadone is a synthetic opioid, it is taken usually by mouth as a green liquid (1 mg/ml) or as a 5 mg tablet. Ampoules of methadone for injection are available (50 mg). Orally it produces little euphoria to the heroin addict, but relieves his physical symptoms and craving over 12–24 hours. As mentioned above, it is used widely as a 'maintenance' treatment to minimise harm; by regular prescription the hypothesis is that the patient will not engage in criminal activities or put his body at risk from harmful activities such as injecting and prostitution. Sadly, many patients who are prescribed methadone in the outpatient community continue to use heroin as well, deepening the tolerance and habituation. Patients on a regular methadone prescription experience worse withdrawal symptoms for longer than those on heroin alone.

Methadone is the traditional drug used in assisting opiate withdrawal by direct substitution, starting with a dose of perhaps 50–60 ml and then steadily weaning off over a variable period of time, perhaps 10–20 days, but often much longer. Various patterns of methadone reduction are favoured by differing treatment centres. I favour none of them. Methadone is very hard to let go of for the opiate addict. The first few days may go smoothly enough, but as the drug is tailed off and for the first few days of abstinence, withdrawals can be severe. This will happen more than a week into treatment by which time the initial wave of motivation will have passed. It is both difficult for a caring treatment team to offer no treatment to a patient in distress, and difficult for the patient to endure; I am certain that patients default from treatment because of this.

Clonidine and lofexidine

Clonidine was originally introduced as a powerful blood pressure lowering drug though is seldom used for this purpose now. It is also occasionally used in low dose to prevent migraine and to treat menopausal hot flushes. It is both a peripheral alpha adrenergic blocking drug, and it has mixed central and sympathomimetic effects — it is these latter effects that we exploit in assisting opiate withdrawal. Although it is not an opiate analogue and does not occupy opiate receptor sites, it partially blocks the excitation, particularly of sympathetic pathways, that opiate withdrawal initiates. It does not ease craving, nor does it have any analgesic action, but it eases the rhinorrhoea, epiphora, hyperasthesia and diaphoretic symptoms of opiate withdrawal. In other words, it helps some of the physical distress while allowing the patient to experience and control his own desire to use heroin.

It does have side effects, it causes a dry mouth, blurred vision, is slightly sedative and, of course, it lowers blood pressure. The hypotensive effects cause the legs to feel leaden, a feeling of light headedness particularly on standing, and faintness. The few occurrences of occulogyric phenomena that I have seen have passed on discontinuation of the drug.

Lofexidine has an identical mode of action to clonidine but was introduced specifically as a drug to aid opiate detoxification. It is less hypotensive than clonidine but I am open minded as to whether it is as effective in easing opiate withdrawals. Lofexidine is regarded as having fewer side-effects than clonidine and its comparative lack of hypotension makes it far more suitable for use in the community. But paradoxically, I think that worse side-effects make clonidine a more attractive drug in residential treatment. Opiate abusers are usually well experienced with large quantities of many different drugs and are immediately sceptical of a drug that they have not tried before, and which has few obvious effects. It is possible to 'talk up' clonidine by dwelling on its powerful effects and, in my view, opiate users are more impressed by a drug that makes them heavy-legged and dizzy when they stand up. Moreover, many opiate addicts coming into residential treatment have already tried and failed community lofexidine, and will have little faith in a second attempt. These reasons for favouring clonidine may sound rather cynical, but I have no doubt that successful opiate detoxification has far more to do with confidence than science.

Both drugs must be initiated slowly and titrated up against the patient's blood pressure and symptoms (see regimen below). They must be withdrawn similarly slowly, to avoid what is known as 'rebound hypertension'.

Naltrexone

Naltrexone is a very powerful opiate antagonist. It is an opiate analogue alleged to have no intrinsic agonist activity which acts by having a very high affinity for opiate receptor sites in the brain, and displaces any other opiate or endorphin from them. It is long acting, a single tablet lasting over 24 hours. It has few side effects, the most notable being anhedonia. It is marketed and licenced as an aid to maintaining abstinence from opiates. A daily tablet will block any effect whatsoever from dosing with almost any amount of heroin or other opiate. It is absolutely contraindicated from being administered to a patient that is actively addicted as by displacing the drug it provokes immediate and profound withdrawals. Despite this manufacturers warning there are some centres that are now offering rapid detoxification under either very heavy sedation, or even anaesthesia, by administering naltrexone to 'wash out' heroin from the brain over perhaps, just a weekend. Although this method may be superficially appealing (certainly to the patient) I do not believe, irrespective of the risks involved, that there is much place for this treatment. Research shows that there is far more to maintaining abstinence than just the relatively mechanistic step of actual withdrawal.

If the patient has invested nothing in his treatment, but simply passed his withdrawal over to the doctor and woken up two days later, then he has invested nothing in his recovery and will have little to loose should he relapse. In fact, after this treatment patients feel very ill indeed, and those who I have seen are prescribed a large number of differing drugs to take over the next week or so. I question what is supposed to have been achieved by this expensive and dangerous treatment?

In the residential setting we have several weeks of the patient's time. A clonidine detox will have the patient opiate free very quickly, is safe and allows the patient to take part in the psychotherapeutic part of the programme quickly.

Buprenorphine

Buprenorphine is becoming a popularly prescribed drug in some countries as a strong pain killer. Notably, in France, it has the same role as methadone in substitution therapy. It is a synthetic opiate that is presented in tablet form, either as a tablet to be swallowed or absorbed buccaly. It is a powerful analgesic, can produce dysphoria or euphoria in large dosage, and has a duration of action of eight hours or so. It is gaining in popularity because it is alleged that it is not so difficult to withdraw from as methadone. Unfortunately, it is readily abused by the tablets being reduced to liquid and then injected. It can also be used in gradual reduction to wean the patient to abstinence in the same way and with the same difficulties as methadone.

Codeine

Codeine is a natural opiate and is the major constituent of raw opium, the second being morphine, and the remainder less important alkaloids. Codeine is widely employed in prescription, and over-the-counter medications, in cough mixtures, diarrhoea medicines and analgesics. There is a more potent ester of codeine, dihydrocodeine that is particularly popular as an analgesic and as a drug of abuse. Codeine addiction is not very common in the UK, though common in France where it is the usual heroin substitution medication. Large doses of codeine are weakly euphoric and for all practical purposes may be treated in the same way as methadone. It has no value whatever in my practice, either for weaning off opiates or in any other role, being 'neither fish nor fowl'.

Loperamide

Loperamide is a powerful anti-diarrhoeal medication that works by acting on the gut's opiate receptors. It is thought to be gut receptor specific and not to have a significant effect on the brain's opiate receptors. That said, in overdosage it does cause CNS depression that is reversible with the opiate antagonist naloxone. It is doubtful whether this drug is of any interest to the opiate abuser and, having treated many such patients, I have only come across one patient who was misusing loperamide. It is of undoubted value in the short term relief of diarrhoea in opiate withdrawals.

Domperidone

Domperidone has little central action, but is an effective anti-emetic by promoting gastric emptying and correcting upper gastro intestinal dysmotility. It can be given as a tablet or suppository. It is safe, has few significant side effects and is the drug of choice in treating vomiting in opiate (or alcohol) withdrawals. Traditional anti-emetics based on phenothiazines are to be avoided if possible, as they offer a sedative 'reward' and can therefore be demanded inappropriately.

Analgesia

It is worth briefly mentioning analgesia in opiate withdrawals. Pain is a very common problem in the patient withdrawing from opiates; the routine stomach cramps, loin pain and general hyperasthesia are to be expected as the pain threshold seeks to self-adjust to an equilibrium when the heavy burden of opiates have been removed. Similarly, old injuries, back problems, dental pain and so forth will become much more painful during detox and for some weeks or even months later. Analgesics 'on demand' will be readily sought by opiate addicts to ease these pains, ease their somatised anxieties and by being available as and when requested, will be the only drugs available to exploit. It is important to adhere rigidly to a policy of giving only simple analgesics that have no central action, which really limits the medical team to paracetamol or non steroidal anti-inflammatory drugs (NSAIDS). These drugs are fairly ineffective at easing pain in opiate withdrawal as the pain is being mediated by opiate receptors that have been vacated, and it is only opiate analogues that will bind to these and be effective in relieving their pain. I always make this explanation to the patient, that their pain is to be expected, that it will lessen in time, and that little can be done pharmaceutically to help. Hot baths, massages with or without aromatherapy oils are all soothing, and I have also employed acupuncture to good effect.

Pregnancy

We are receiving a small but increasing number of women who are seeking treatment for opiate addiction during pregnancy. Opiate addiction itself carries an increased risk of miscarriage, introduces difficulties of analgesia for the mother in childbirth, and results in an opiate addicted infant that needs special nursing in its early days of life while going through its own withdrawal syndrome. Clearly it is desirable to detoxify the mother (and foetus) during early pregnancy to avoid these complications. In my experience there are no special difficulties here. The risk of miscarriage is no higher than if the pregnancy were to continue, and there is no evidence of foetal harm from the medications that we use. It is rational that distress to the pregnancy should be minimal so there is clear medical justification for the detoxification to be made as slowly and comfortably as possible.

Stimulants and others

This section concerns a disparate group of drugs which I am simply classing together for convenience. In order of importance by virtue of numbers through treatment, these are:

- cocaine and crack cocaine
- amphetamine sulphate
- methylenedioxymethamphetamine — MDMA (Ecstasy)
- LSD
- sundries, ie. dexedrine, benzedrine, ritalin etc.

Cocaine

This drug has become much more commonly used outside South America over recent decades, and with the advent of its alkalated derivative 'Crack' cocaine, its use has exploded the world over. Although cocaine remains the more exotic 'party' drug for the rich and famous, crack, which is intensely psychologically addictive, is less expensive and has been connected to organised criminal activity and to the poorer and more disadvantaged sectors of society.

Cocaine comes from the leaves of the coco plant of South America, where it has been chewed by local people for centuries, for its restorative and stimulating properties. Pure cocaine powder is absorbed rapidly over mucous membranes, and the chosen route is to inhale it nasally, either out of a tiny spoon, or through a rolled up card off a hard surface such as a mirror, where it has been divided into 'lines'. It can also be taken between gum and lip, vaginally, rectally, or under the foreskin where its local anaesthetic action may have the side effect of delaying ejaculation. It becomes effective within a few minutes, causing euphoria, elation, energy and disinhibition. The effect lasts up to an hour or so initially, but tolerance develops rapidly and the duration of action becomes shorter. Crack cocaine is a rough crystalline substance made by introducing bicarbonate or ammonia to a saturated aqueous solution of cocaine, the drug precipitating as large lumps of crystals. While some people like to 'freebase' their own crack in this way, it is usually bought as the 'rock' product that is smoked in small pipes or adapted soft drink cans. Crack cocaine produces a very rapid and intense excitation which diminishes rapidly after only a few minutes. The rapid depletion causes cravings and an insatiable greed for more drug. It is very difficult for the user to put any of his supply down and, once started, the binge usually continues until the supply (and the user's money) are all consumed.

However, unlike opiates the body experiences little in the way of withdrawal symptoms from cocaine apart from exhaustion and some depression. The pattern for some users is to buy the drug at the end of the week when they receive pay, 'party' all weekend then return to work on Monday. Others prefer to smoke crack as often as they can raise the funds to buy it, to the exclusion of all else. It becomes an obsession at the expense of work and relationships. Some heroin users like to mix either cocaine or crack cocaine with heroin and inject it, when supplies are available. Equally, cocaine users frequently abuse other chemicals to wind down after a heavy binge, so that they can sleep and recuperate from what can be a very exhausting time. Alcohol may serve this purpose, also quenching thirst and being binged in enormous amounts while partying. Cocaine users frequently adopt a rather superior attitude over heroin users, but some may smoke heroin to come down from a binge, a heroin addiction subsequently starting in this way.

Cocaine and crack cocaine are very stimulating, encouraging activity and diminishing the body's ability to perceive exhaustion, hence users have boundless energy to work, dance etc. Consequently, many users appear to be very fit, lean and muscular.

For reasons that are not clear to me they also often have quite bad acne that soon clears with abstinence. Of course, injecting cocaine exposes the user to all the risks mentioned under injecting opiates, although, in purely physical terms harm from the drug itself is relatively limited. The principle risk comes from the extreme stress that these drugs subject the cardiovascular system to, and sudden death from acute cardiac disrythmias and internal haemorrhage may occur, although this is not common

On the other hand, harm to the patient's mental and social health is enormous. Personality change is profound and affects all who use cocaine, at first temporarily, but subsequently in a more pervasive way. Initially the user may seem confident, genial and fun to be with, but with regular use the typical cocaine user often becomes obnoxious, overbearing, unreliable and generally a rather odious person to be with. Work colleagues may notice the user being extremely energetic and focused on his task, yet producing poor quality work. Paranoia is common and frank psychosis affects many users at times. This psychosis is usually reversible with abstinence but may be longer lasting. Relationships frequently suffer and breakdown of family is commonplace.

The amphetamines

Amphetamines are sometimes considered the poor man's cocaine, though there are some who make it their drug of choice above all others. Amphetamines were discovered many years ago, and have been used in medicine for a long time, usually in frivolous ways. For instance, benzedrine was prescribed by the Royal Navy to night watch officers on ships to keep them awake, and other amphetamine analogues have been widely prescribed to aid weight loss. It is only in relatively recent years in the UK that they have even been classed as controlled substances and, all but a few, withdrawn. Large quantities are still available abroad both from medical suppliers and illegal manufacturing sources.

The most widely abused amphetamine is amphetamine sulphate, or dexamphetamine sulphate. This is supplied in powder form and can be taken in just about any way: it can be inhaled through the nose as a powder, smoked in a joint, injected or swallowed. It causes stimulation and excitation, probably in excess of cocaine, but is less euphoric. The effect of a single dose may be felt for up to ten hours, depending on the route of administration and tolerance. Ecstasy is a tablet preparation of an amphetamine analogue which more closely mimics cocaine in that it is more euphoric and less stimulating than plain amphetamine. There must be important differences in the quality of experience as, without exception, all the users that I have spoken to who have used both, would always prefer cocaine. Ecstasy is however very cheap.

The harm profile of the amphetamines is much the same as that of cocaine. There have been several tragic and well published sudden deaths in apparently fit young people who have experimented with Ecstasy. The exact cause of these deaths is not entirely understood and may indeed be multifactorial. Certainly, these drugs are prepared by unskilled pharmacists with no quality control and may well be contaminated by more toxic substances that are incidental to the manufacture. Additionally, it is felt that some deaths are caused by acute electrolyte imbalances brought on by dehydration (or paradoxically over hydration) as the drugs are used to stimulate tireless dancing for many hours in very hot rooms.

The hallucinogens

It seems that almost every week a new hallucinogen is manufactured by some backstreet laboratory, yet the hallucinogen that has stood the test of time par excellence, is LSD (lysergic acid diethylamide).

LSD has been in widespread use since the early 1960s. It is usually taken orally as a small tablet, or a piece of blotting paper that the drug has been absorbed onto. The effects begin within half an hour, and last about nine hours. It is an exceedingly powerful hallucinogen, distorting perception of what is real and introducing vivid fantasies into the conscious, and all senses, especially sight, but also sound, taste and touch. The effects can be magical and wondrous, but because of their intensity, they can also be terrifying.

Tolerance develops after a single dose, it is almost impossible to derive benefit from LSD for two days running because the neurotransmitters that it modulates are all washed out by the first dose, and it takes a few days for them to replenish. There is therefore no 'dependency' to LSD, although many individuals use it on a recurring basis because they enjoy it so much.

I am not aware of any direct physical harm particular to LSD. It completely disables logic, judgement and a sense of self-preservation until it wears off, so users are sometimes in grave peril if they attempt to drive a car or swim, and most cases of physical harm arise accidentally. We have all heard of cases of individuals jumping out of windows, believing that they can fly, or perhaps trying to hold a conversation with cars on a motorway, with disastrous consequences. The mental harm is as much as it is for cocaine and amphetamines. Personality changes, paranoia and drug induced psychosis can be profound, occasionally long lasting. In the case of LSD, some play is made of 'flashbacks' where without provocation an individual may suddenly experience hallucinations from years before. I think this must be rare because although most drug users I speak to believe that this happens, none have said that it has it actually happened to them.

Treatment

These patients pose little work for the medical arm of the treatment team; they are often very fit and experience little, if any, physical withdrawal symptoms. A 'crash' or series of crashes is to be anticipated in some individuals after heavy or prolonged use, where the patient becomes extremely tired and needs a long period of sleep, sometimes several days. There is no reason why the patient should not take part in the programme at this time, they can be woken and encouraged to meetings, but they may doze off and make little contribution for a few days. Later on in treatment a few patients become depressed and some treatment centres advocate the use of tricyclic antidepressants. I do not: I have never seen profound depression in stimulant users that was not transitory or responsive to the psychotherapeutic approach. I do, however, offer sedation over three days to facilitate the sleeping off period.

As with all patients, the doctor should see the patient as soon as possible after admission; the history and examination is as for opiate or alcohol users. There are no physical conditions particular to stimulant users that the physician should look out for, except perhaps the universally dreadful sounding chest in the crack smoker, and damaged nareal mucosa of the cocaine or amphetamine sniffer. Most of these signs resolve within the first three weeks of abstinence. Once I saw mitral leaflet prolapse in a man who had used large amounts of amphetamine daily for many years so that he could work for 16 hours daily and then play two hours of squash afterwards. He had literally torn his cardiac papillary muscles apart.

Opiate detoxification protocol

Clonidine

Clonidine is my preferred drug for easing the physical symptoms of opiate withdrawal. Because it is such a powerful drug in lowering blood pressure, the dose needs to be weaned on over two to three days to minimise the risk of hypotensive episodes; and weaned off over two to three days at the end of the treatment period, to minimise the risk of rebound hypertension.

Inevitably, the first two days of clonidine treatment are inadequate at the time when the patient's symptoms will be at their worst. It is reasonable to bridge this gap with methadone if the patient (as happens almost invariably) requests it. If patients are already on an out- patient methadone prescription I like them to arrive in treatment having taken their day's dose of methadone. This covers the first day of clonidine introduction. The second day, as the dose of clonidine is increasing, I give half their usual methadone daily allowance, and by the third day they will be on adequate clonidine and no further methadone is given. If they are not used to methadone, ie. they are using heroin alone, a small dose of methadone, say 20 mg, is sufficient on the second day. If the patient is being detoxified from a different opiate, such as codeine or buprenorphine, it may be preferable to use their drug of choice in half dose on the second day, instead of methadone.

The dosage schedule given below is for guidance and is not intended to be prescriptive. The aim is to give as much clonidine as the patient's blood pressure can safely take. The patient's blood pressure must be taken before every dosage and should be as much a guide as their symptoms. If they are handling their withdrawal symptoms fairly well there is no pressure to increase clonidine any further. On the other hand, if there is evidence of discomfort, rhinorrhoea etc and they have no symptoms of dizziness, faintness and so forth when standing, the dose may be increased further.

In addition to clonidine, I also prescribe a small dose of the benzodiazepine oxazepam for the first four nights in patients who are not to receive benzodiazepines for other reasons (ie. concurrent alcohol or benzodiazepine detoxification). I accept that there is no compelling reason for this and do not suggest that this is mandatory. However, it is only for four nights and it is something 'extra' to give confidence to the patient who is fearful of the withdrawal process.

Day:	1	2	3	4	5	6	7	8	9	10
Methadone	*	**	0	0	0	0	0	0	0	0
Oxazepam (mg. nocte)	30	30	30	30	0	0	0	0	0	0
Clonidine (mg in 24 hrs) (see nursing notes below)	0.3	0.6	0.8	0.8	0.8	0.8	0.8	0.8	0.6	0.4
OR:										
Lofexidine (mg in 24 hrs)	0.6	1.0	1.4	1.8	1.8	1.8	1.8	1.4	1.0	0.1

(**Note** methadone: * = the patient should have already taken his daily allowance prior to admission, so methadone is not normally administered on the day of admission. In any event, it is impossible to know exactly what he may have used having just arrived at the treatment centre — further opiate dosing may cause overdosage.
**=give half their previous daily allowance divided into two separate doses, or 20 mg total if the patient is not normally taking methadone, ie. using heroin alone.)

Nursing notes

Patients should be counselled regarding the symptoms of hypotension, and advised against rapid rising from the chair or bed, or vigorous exertion.

The first dose of clonidine needs to be given as soon as possible, it is desirable to get as much clonidine in the first day as time allows. The first dose is a 'test' dose of 0.1 mg as patients' blood pressure response to clonidine is variable. The patient must be instructed to return after an hour for a blood pressure check. Unusually there may be a sharp drop in blood pressure of 15 mm Hg systolic and this must be reported to the doctor. In most cases there will have been less effect on blood pressure and thereafter dosage of clonidine is repeated six to eight hourly working within the guidelines above. The blood pressure and pulse must be taken and recorded before each dose. The patient's symptoms are actually more important than the blood pressure alone; many patients are accustomed to normally low blood pressure and symptoms of dizziness and faintness are more important than the absolute recording. Such symptoms should be responded to by checking the blood pressure with the patient standing as well as sitting, and a systolic blood pressure of 85 mm Hg or less must be reported to the doctor as soon as possible, as should any unusual symptoms or concerns. Hypotension should be treated by putting the patient to bed and raising the foot of the bed. The doctor's advice should then be sought.

In the event of serious hypotension it may be possible to change over to lofexidine, or continue clonidine at a lower dose, perhaps with additional oxazepam sedation.

Methadone reduction

This is being described for information purposes only. I do not favour methadone weaning, but there is occasional place for it, for instance in patients for whom clonidine is contraindicated.

There is no special formula for reducing methadone, it beomes progressively more uncomfortable for the patient as the dose decreases. In the residential setting, we are keen to remove all medication as soon as possible and to reduce methadone by 5 mg per day is reasonable, although poorly tolerated.

Pregnancy

The pregnant patient should have sought approval for detoxification from her obstetrician, prior to her admission. There should be no antenatal complications and the community midwife should be involved at an early stage.

Clonidine and lofexidine are not sanctioned by their manufacturers for use in pregnancy but, in my opinion, they may be used in the second and third trimesters with the patient's informed consent, the greatest worry being placental insufficiency through prolonged hypotension.

A balance needs to be struck between too distressing a detox, with the attendant risk of miscarriage or premature labour, and hypotension. My advice is to give lofexidine at a lower dose, perhaps half the dose given in the schedules above, and to aim to keep the systolic blood pressure above 95 mm Hg for as much of the treatment period as possible. The lesser dose of lofexidine will obviously have a lesser control of withdrawal symptoms and so it is reasonable in the pregnant patient to concurrently administer small and reducing doses of methadone for the first four to six days.

Detoxifying the pregnant opiate addict is not unduly difficult, but may be best carried out in those centres that are experienced in this field.

Accelerated lofexidine regime

Bearn *et al* (1998) describe a novel course of lofexidine, beginning with high doses and reducing over five days (see *Table 11*). The results on patients' symptom scores compare very favourably with the conventional ten day course given above. I have no experience of administering this regime but respect the author's view that this may offer more immediate symptom relief and allow earlier participation in the rehabilitation programme. The work also underscores the safety of lofexidine so far as hypotension is concerned and, by implication, that the weaning on phase of the conventional ten day regime is probably an unnecessary caution.

Table 11: Accelerated lofexidine regime						
Day	1	2	3	4	5	6
Dose (mg) frequency	0.6 3x	1 2x	1 2x	1 2x	0.6 2x	0
Total (mg) in 24 hrs	1.8	2	2	2	1.2	0

Reference

Bearn J, Glossop M, Strang J (1998) Accelerated lofexidine. *Drug Alcohol Depend* **50**: 227–232

Alcohol detoxification protocol

Chlordiazepoxide and diazepam

Either of these are used to reduce the stress to the nervous system as a substitute sedative to ethanol that can be controllably weaned off over a few days. Signs of CNS excitation are tremors, sweating, tachycardia and raised blood pressure. These drugs are extremely safe, even in doses several times higher than could ever be needed. The only risks from over dosage are undesirably excessive sedation, with the attendant risk of accidental harm from falls. The dose may begin high and be reduced quite quickly so that almost all patients should be off sedation in five to seven days.

Carbamazepine

This is my drug of choice in reducing the risk of epileptiform withdrawal seizures. It is given at a dose of 200 mg twice daily until sedation (chlordiazepoxide) is discontinued, then 100 mg twice daily for a further five days. Carbamazepine is itself a sedative, and has dose related toxic effects upon liver and bone marrow. This dose schedule is a compromise between desired anti-convulsant effect and undesirable side-effects. It is important for staff and patient alike to understand that the risk of seizure cannot be eliminated altogether. Fits may very rarely occur during or after completion of carbamazepine, but this schedule affords a good margin of safety with a reasonably brief period of sedation.

Pabrinex

I prefer the intramuscular preparation of this high potency vitamin supplement, to pre-empt Wernicke's encephalopathy. The injections come as pairs of ampoules, are painful and should be given deep intramuscularly, once to twice daily for up to five days.

Notes to nurses

Remember that sedation is administered to achieve safety, not comfort. Inevitably, these patients will be anxious and this anxiety will be gratifyingly eased by the sedation. But the priority is to reduce the stress to the **whole** nervous system and this is objectively assessed by examining the patient for tremor, sweating, raised blood pressure and pulse.

On admission patients may very well be intoxicated, sometimes severely. Such patients should be put to bed and monitored at least half hourly. They should be placed on their sides in 'the recovery position', and have their conscious level, pulse, blood pressure and urine output monitored. Any signs of deterioration should be reported to the doctor **immediately**.

As the patient's intoxication wears off he should be encouraged to get up and mix with his peers who can be your extra 'eyes and ears'. The patient must report back frequently in the early stages of admission, and less frequently over the next few days. On each occasion the pulse and blood pressure should be taken and the patient's overall condition assessed. Attention should be paid to complaints of blurred vision, double vision or other visual disturbance, ataxia, and paradoxical depression of conscious state.

The question arises as to what dose of chlordiazepoxide or diazepam should be given at any one time, it being left totally to the discretion of the nursing team. As has been stated, the purpose of sedation is to reduce the stress to the nervous system as evidenced by rises in blood pressure and pulse rate, sweating, withdrawal seizures and even hallucinations. The risk of overdosing does not come from the drug itself, but from masking clouding of consciousness, which may be caused by intracranial bleeds or impending encephalopathy.

The risks from alcohol withdrawal reduce exponentially with time and I prefer frequent small doses rather than less frequent large lumps of sedation. In this way the patient will be under frequent review by the nursing team, and his condition will be subtly adjusted as appropriate. This will minimise the risk of missing deteriorating consciousness and confine the total amount of sedation to the minimum necessary.

Accordingly, except under quite exceptional circumstances, most patients can be managed with doses of chlordiazepoxide 40 mg or diazepam 15 mg, totalling less than chlordiazepoxide 280 mg or diazepam 100 mg in the first 24 hours.

Typical alcohol detoxification regime										
Day:	1	2	3	4	5	6	7	8	9	10
Chlordiaze-poxide (mg in 24 hrs)	140	80	20	20	0	0	0	0	0	0
Carbamazepine 400 (mg in 24 hrs)	400	400	400	400	200	200	200	200	200	0
Pabrinex IMM (pairs ampoules intramuscularly)	1	1	1	1	1	0	0	0	0	0

(**Notes:** This is an illustration, dosages will vary widely (see text). On day 1 a little sedation may be needed if the patient arrives late and intoxicated.)

Stimulants detoxification protocol

As there is no appreciable physical withdrawal state from stimulants, there is no specific need for medication to assist withdrawal. Indeed, many patients use stimulants on a bingeing pattern and are well used to periods of being drug free. That said, there are some, particularly amphetamine users, who use the drug in large amounts, perhaps intravenously, every day for years. Abrupt withdrawal is a terrifying prospect to some and provokes intense cravings. It must be remembered that they will be admitted alongside alcohol and heroin abusers who will be given medication and inevitably they may feel aggrieved at being given no drug assistance whatsoever.

It is reasonable, although arguably so, to offer a brief reduction regime of mild sedation to ease cravings and anxiety. I prefer oxazepam, if only because it has some cachet in that most drug abusers have not heard of it. But, since it has such a specious role, I would not argue with any suitable replacement.

In fact most stimulant users become extremely tired soon after admission and frequently spend up to 48 hours in bed, mostly asleep.

Oxazepam protocol for stimulant withdrawal
Day:
1} 2}   oxazepam 30 mg three times daily
3} 4}   oxazepam 15 mg twice daily and 30 mg at night
5} 6}   oxazepam 30 mg at night

Benzodiazepine detoxification protocol

This schedule is also appropriate for barbiturate and meprobamate. At the risk of generalising, there are two distinct profiles of benzodiazepine user:

* the heroin addict who regularly uses illicitly acquired benzodiazepines, typically diazepam or temazepam in wildly variable amounts according to availability, either intravenously or orally and,

* the patient who has been prescribed benzodiazepines, usually diazepam or lorazepam, for many years by the medical profession.

This latter patient may also abuse alcohol, with or without physical dependency. Both sets of patient by definition are used to medicating away their feelings of anxiety and are inevitably extremely anxious about giving up their drug. And well they might be, because benzodiazepine withdrawal is characterised by severe rebound anxiety, restlessness, panic attacks and insomnia. There is no simple way to escape this inevitable pattern, all that can be achieved is as slow a weaning off as is practicable.

There is no point in using large numbers of different benzodiazepines in a treatment centre, it is as well to get familiar with one or two and stick to them. They all have near identical effects, and indeed most have common active metabolites. The main practical differences are in potency, duration of action and 'attack rates'.

I favour converting the patient's typical use into an equipotent dose of diazepam (see *Table 7, page 21*) and then weaning this off over a period of two to four weeks, according to the amount and duration of use. The rate that the dose diminishes should taper off exponentially. The diazepam should be offered to the patient as daily rations, to be given in divided doses, leaving him to take less by day and more at night to assist sleeping if he so chooses. It is **absolutely vital** to prepare the patient for this process, preferably before he even arrives in the treatment centre, to set the boundaries, explain supportively that a degree of rebound anxiety is unavoidable, and that no doses will be increased or held **under any circumstances**.

Carbamazepine is used to prevent seizures in the same way as for alcohol withdrawal. It is mandatory for any patient who has experienced seizures before, and advisable for patients who have used large amounts of benzodiazepines for a number of years.

Example of a reduction in a patient who has been using benzodiazepines for many years, currently the equivalent dose of 100 mg diazepam:

Day	1	2	3	4	5	6	7			
Diazepam (mg) 100	90	80	75	70	65	60	55			
Day	**8**	**9**	**10**	**11**	**12**	**13**	**14**			
Diazepam (mg)	50	45	40	35	30	25	20			
Day	**15**	**16**	**17**	**18**	**19**	**20**	**21**	**22**	**23**	**24**
Diazepam (mg)	18	16	14	12	10	8	6	4	2	

Other drugs and non drug treatments

Domperidone

This is a useful non-sedating anti-emetic. It may be given in severe cases of vomiting as a rectal suppository in a dose of 30 mg, or as a 10 mg tablet. The usual dose is orally 10–20 mg every six to eight hours, or rectally, 30 mg every eight hours, as required.

Loperamide

This is an effective anti-diarrhoeal and may be used to treat the diarrhoea that usually occurs in the early stages of opiate withdrawals. It is given as an oral 2 mg capsule, every six hours if required. It should not be needed for more than two to three days.

Laxatives

There is little if any need for aperients on a regular basis and requests should alert suspicion of an eating disorder. Appropriate dosages are:

> lactulose syrup 10–20 ml twice daily or,
>
> fybogel one sachet in water twice daily.

Both of these are safe to give limitlessly and will not be abused by those with eating disorders as they cause abdominal gaseous distension.

Analgesics

These are often requested to ease the pains of opiate withdrawals, or other pains, notably headaches, which may well be somatised anxiety. Requests should always be critically examined. Our patients have a habit of medicating away unpleasant feelings and they need to be reminded that trivial requests for analgesics are lesser examples of the same behaviour. Most headaches pass soon enough and there should be a constant 'downward pressure' on the issue of these medications, not so much because the drugs themselves are harmful, but because the behaviour may be.

For the opiate addict in pain, only opiates will work. Clearly these may not be given 'as required'; the patients must be reassured that their pain thresholds will normalise as treatment progresses. For the normal aches and pains:

paracetomol 500 mg tabs, two to be taken every eight hours, or

ibuprofen 400 mg every eight hours.

Naltrexone

This drug (see *pages 33–34*) may be of infrequent use. Patients who have completed their opiate detoxification, who are to leave treatment prematurely for whatever reason, and who state that they wish to remain abstinent pending further treatment or completion of their programme, may be offered naltrexone to help keep their recovery safe over a short period of a few weeks or so. Given as a daily tablet, preferably witnessed, it will completely block the effects of opiates, should they relapse. They must be warned however (as must all patients leaving teatment after opiate withdrawal) that their tolerance to opiates has also been withdrawn, and should they relapse without taking naltrexone, they will be at grave risk of overdose that may be fatal.

Acupuncture

I have no idea how acupuncture works, and remain to be convinced that it ever 'cures' anyone of anything. However, I am certain that it can and does ease some of the distressing feelings in withdrawal from chemical addiction, especially anxiety, insomnia and the generalised pains of opiate withdrawals. Various experts with far more experience of this medical art than I will be able to expound more competently, but needling the following points two or three times over ten days or so, is enormously beneficial to some patients, especially those whose motivation has nearly expired and who may default from treatment without further support. The points are:

S–7, Li–4, H–7, S–44, Sp–8

Appendix I

Eating disorders

There are many interesting and expert works on anorexia and bulimia nervosa for the reader to refer to, but I feel a brief mention should be made here because these problems are frequently encountered during the treatment of addiction.

Sometimes an eating disorder is overt and the patient readily admits to either a past or current history. Frequently, however, such disorders become apparent although denied by the patient. The patient is usually a female heroin addict, although it should be remembered that men can be affected and that eating disorders are more common in all types of addiction because the roots of both may arise from distortions in emotional development. The psycho-therapeutic aims of treatment will be the same, but it is important for the patient to identify his/her eating disorder openly.

It might be assumed that an eating disorder is quite easy to identify, but among chemical abusers it most certainly is not. Sufferers of bulimia may be of normal weight or even overweight and, of course, many alcohol and heroin abusers are poorly nourished because of years of self-neglect rather than deliberate starvation. Furthermore, the discomfort of detoxification may cause nausea, vomiting, and an understandable reluctance to eat, so although an eating disorder is frequently suspected, it is usually very difficult or even impossible to prove. Requests for aperients may alert suspicion as purging is frequently associated with anorexia. I prefer to give bulking agents such as Ispagula Husk for such requests since it will assist the genuinely constipated yet by causing bulking and flatus in the colon, have the opposite of the desired effect in the anorexic. If body mass is dangerously low, a contract with the patient must be entered into where if they continue to loose weight they may be discharged from treatment. It is important to be supportive and to ally oneself to the patient by stating that it is not our intention to make him/her fat, merely to keep safe from harmful malnutrition. Controlled self-starvation is as much an addiction as any that we treat. It is essential for successful treatment of the whole patient that this is identified by the patient and included in her/his aim for recovery

Solvents

The availability and cheapness of solvents means that they are widely abused irregularly by schoolchildren as well as being the chemical of choice for a few adults, sometimes in large amounts. Butane, volatile adhesives, and cleaning products are sometimes used in vast quantities on a daily basis, often associated with alcohol abuse. They offer the user near instant intoxication through stupor to unconsciousness. These chemicals are dangerous; quite apart from the fire hazard that they represent, they render the user incapable or unconscious and thus at high risk from aspirating vomit or asphyxiation in the polythene bag that contains the solvent which is often used to inhale the vapours from. There are many accidental deaths each year from these causes. In the long term, organic chemical sovents are toxic to the liver and the central nervous system, indeed, more so than alcohol.

If an abuser seeks our treatment and is using these chemicals in large amounts on a daily basis they can, for the purposes of medically assisted withdrawal, be considered as sedatives and the patient is easily withdrawn with the aid of a few days weaning sedation.

Cannabis

The plant Cannabis Sativa provides leaves, resin and pollen, all of which contain tetra hydro canabinol (THC), the plant's main pschoactive drug. Usually smoked alone in dried leaf form (grass, ganja, keef) or as the resin (hash) with tobacco, cannabis can also be eaten. A variety with a particularly high concentration of THC and a pungent aroma known as 'skunk' has become available. Cannabis is the most widely used illicit recreational drug in the world after tobacco and alcohol. Considering how widely it is used and over so many centuries, it is perhaps surprising that so many myths surround it. It produces a sense of warmth, well being, sedation and to a lesser degree, elation and distortion of perception. Trivial tasks can become impossibly difficult and preposterous. It may also stimulate the appetite and cause short term difficulties with memory. There is little, if any, evidence of a physical withdrawal syndrome, and similarly slight evidence of physical harm although inhaling the fumes of burning vegetable matter does not have a good record of safety (*qv.* tobacco). Modest occasional use of cannabis appears to be relatively harmless.

However as with alcohol, cannabis has the potential for abuse. It is widely used by those who abuse heroin, cocaine and other illicit drugs, and some individuals become obsessed with consuming enormous quantities of cannabis. In these circumstances it is socially harmful, and psychologically leads to personality changes and paranoia. There is no physical withdrawal state and craving can be eased with a little oxazepam if it is deemed desirable. It is included in our intent for abstinence from all mind affecting chemicals because it disinhibits and frequently initiates the slide back into relapse from more important addictions.

Polydrug abuse

I never cease to be amazed by the variety and quantity of drugs that some individuals are capable of surviving on a regular basis. Of course, many claims are exaggerated either through bravado or an attempt to negotiate a 'generous' detox, but there are many who undeniably will try anything and everything that is available to them. It is near impossible to obtain an accurate history as their stories are invariably unreliable, either because of misrepresentation or because, having consumed so much, they have no recollection of what they have actually been doing. Therefore, it might seem that prescribing an appropriate detox in this situation is very difficult.

It is not. For practical purposes there are only three chemicals that require medical assistance in withdrawal: alcohol, opiates and sedatives. So far as opiates are concerned it does not matter how much or what type as all are subject to the same detox with clonidine. Similarly alcohol, if drunk daily, will be subject to the standard detox as described elsewhere. Finally sedatives (usually benzodiazepines), may probably be withdrawn more quickly than with those for whom it is the drug of choice, as the chaotic drug abuser will be accustomed to variable amounts and periods without. Any other drugs, stimulants and so forth will have their withdrawal catered for by the medication that will be prescribed for the three main groups.

Selective serotonin reuptake inhibiting (SSRI) antidepressants

We are seeing an increasing number of patients arriving in treatment on prescibed antidepressants, usually SSRIs. Members of this new class of drugs are being enthusiastically prescribed by the medical profession because of their efficacy and relative freedom from toxicity and side effects.

On the whole I am sympathetic to this enthusiasm; SSRIs are safe in overdose, saving many deaths from deliberate self- poisoning with the older tricyclic drugs. In addition, because of their lack of undesirable side effects such as sedation, dry mouth, blurred vision, prostatism and so forth, patients are more willing to comply with treatment. Finally, there can be no higher endorsement than their lack of uptake as a drug of illicit use. There are reported cases of the odd Prozac changing hands illegally, but to the main body of drug abusers these drugs have little or no appeal.

There are two principle notes of caution: firstly, some SSRIs are quite anxiolytic, notably paroxetine, and this drug has a now accepted withdrawal syndrome of rebound anxiety and insomnia, and should be withdrawn slowly. Additionally, as has been mentioned, the vast majority of antidepressants are prescribed for reactive depression and it is the the objective of the psychotherapeutic arm of treatment to have our patients respond appropriately to the vicissitudes of everyday life, not to have their emotional responses artificially modulated by any drug, be it legal or illegal. Accordingly, except in cases where there is overwhelming evidence for an organic basis for depression, we would withdraw these drugs during primary treatment.

Appendix II

Glossary of street slang in drug misuse

Street slang is both regional and ephemoral, this list is just a sample.

Acid	LSD
Amps	Ampoules, usually methadone
Ascorbic acid (vit c)	used to dissolve heroin
Bag	small dose of heroin
Banging up	injecting heroin
Billy	amphetamine
Blotters	form of LSD
Blow	cannabis
Blues	barbiturates
Bombs	any pills
Booting	smoking heroin
Bones	crack cocaine
Bong	water pipe to smoke cannabis
Brain	amphetamine
Brown	heroin
Buds	cannabis
Buzz(ing)	effect of a drug
Carrying	in possession of drugs
Charlie	cocaine
Chas	cocaine
Chasing (the dragon)	smoking, usually heroin or crack cocaine

Chewies	Tuinal (barbiturate)
Chillom	pipe to smoke cannabis
Chilling	giving time for a drug to wear off
China white	heroin
Citrate	used to make heroin soluble to inject
Clucking	heroin withdrawal symptoms
Coach and Horses	cocktail of cocaine and heroin
Cold turkey	extreme heroin withdrawal symptoms
Crack	crack cocaine
Cranking	injecting heroin
Cutting	diluting a drug, usually heroin
Dave	cocaine (as in Chas and Dave)
Dennis the Menace	Ecstasy
Dirt	heroin
Dope	usually cannabis but sometimes heroin
Doves	Ecstasy
Downers	tranquillisers, usually valium etc
Es	Ecstasy
Elephants	Ecstasy
Filters	used in preparing heroin injection
Fixing	injecting, usually heroin
Fizz	citric acid, to make heroin soluble for injection
Foil	tin foil to smoke heroin on
Freebasing	making your own crack from cocaine

Ganja	cannabis (West Indian/Rasta name)
Gear	heroin (most popular name)
Go-fast	amphetamine
Gouching (out)	drug induced stupor
Grass	cannabis plant dried leaves
Guns	syringes
H	heroin
Hash	cannabis resin
Henry	heroin
Hit	effect of a drug
Horse	heroin
Jack and Jills	any pills but often LSD
Jacking up	injecting, usually heroin
Jellies	temazepam capsules
Joint	roll up cigarette containing cannabis or heroin
Jonesing	withdrawal symptoms from heroin
Kef or Kif	cannabis (African name)
Kit	amphetamine
Linctus	Methadone
Line	a dose of cocaine, usually sniffed
Macdonalds	Ecstasy
Mixing the gravy	preparing heroin for injection

Necking	swallowing
Nasty	heroin
Olive oil	foil, to smoke heroin on
Paste	amphetamine
Peachies	Palfium (synthetic opioid tablet)
Pinkies	Diconal (synthetic opioid tablet)
Pins	hypodermic needles
Pipe	to smoke crack cocaine usually, or cannabis or heroin
Popping	swallowing pills
Popping, skin	injecting into muscle (no veins left)
Puff	cannabis
Putty	amphetamine
Rattling	withdrawal symptoms (from heroin)
Rhubarb and custard	Ecstasy
Roach	filter in a joint
Roasting	withdrawal symptoms from heroin
Rocks	crack cocaine
Rush	initial effect of a drug
Scoobies	valium
Scoring	obtaining a fresh supply of drug
Script	prescription
Shit	usually cannabis but can be heroin
Skag	heroin (especially in the north of England)

Skins	cigarette papers for rolling joints
Skin popping	injecting into muscle (when no veins left)
Skunk	a strong form of cannabis
Smack	heroin
Spanners	syringes
Speed	amphetamine
Speed ball	cocaine and heroin cocktail
Spliff	roll up cigarette containing cannabis
Spoon	used to prepare heroin for injection
Stones	crack cocaine
Strawberries	Ecstasy
Toot(ing)	smoking, usually heroin
Tots	LSD
Tranx	tranquillisers
Trip	euphoric state usually with LSD or Ecstasy
Turkey	extreme heroin withdrawal symptoms
Whizz	amphetamine
Weed	cannabis
Works	paraphernalia for injecting heroin
Window pains	LSD
Wrap	small dose of heroin
XTC	Ecstasy
Yin Yangs	LSD